Essentials in Hospice Palliative Care Workbook Study Guide for Nurses

Katherine Murray

RN, BSN, MA, CHPCN(C)

Life and Death Matters

Saanichton BC

2010

Essentials in Hospice Palliative Care Workbook

Study Guide for Nurses

by Katherine Murray
RN, BSN, MA, CHPCN(C)

Published by Life and Death Matters, 2958 Lamont Road, Saanichton, BC Canada, V8M 1W5
www.lifeanddeathmatters.ca

Editing and Production by Ann-Marie Gilbert
Design by Ann-Marie Gilbert.
Original Cover: The Noblet Design Group, Regina, Saskatchewan

Library and Archives Canada Cataloguing in Publication
Murray, Katherine, 1957-
Essentials in Hospice Palliative Care. Workbook: Study Guide for Nurses / Katherine Murray
Previously published under title: Essentials in Hospice Palliative Care Workbook.

Includes bibliographical references.
20089076826
ISBN: 978-0973982824
R726.8 M8672 2008
616'.029 22

1. Palliative treatment. 2. Hospice care. 3. Terminal care

Disclaimer

This book is intended to be only a resource of general education on the subject matter. Every effort has been taken to ensure the accuracy of its information, however, there is no guarantee the information will remain current as time extends past the publication date. The information and techniques offered in this book should be used in consultation with qualified medical health professionals and should not be considered a replacement, substitute, or alternative for their guidance, assessment, or treatment. The author and publisher does not accept responsibility or liability to any person or entity with respect to loss or damage or any other problem caused or alleged to be caused directly or indirectly by information contained in this book

About the Cover

The arbutus tree, Canada's only native broadleaf evergreen, grows along the windblown Pacific coast, often on rock bluffs or in rocky soil. The Arbutus tree thrives where no others venture. This gnarled tree, with its eczema-like reddish-brown bark peeling off in papery flakes each spring, stands as a symbol of strength, commitment, perseverance, determination and survival, amidst so many adversities. In these ways, the Arbutus tree symbolizes the strength, beauty, and uniqueness of the human spirit and our ability to grow in the midst of suffering; and to live fully, even in the face of death and dying.

Christine Piercy writes, "The arbutus tree represents that place between life and death, often perched precariously at the meeting place of land and ocean. So it is with those who are dying and those who care for them, as the dying hover in this place of transition between life and death. Those of us who encircle them may long to bring them back into life, or wish that death would take them from this intensely painful place of 'in-between'. Is it possible that, like the Arbutus tree, there can be growth and beauty in such a place?"

Introduction to the Workbook

My goal for Life and Death Matters is to develop resources that will provide caregivers with the "essentials" to provide excellent care for people who are dying. I am aware that when I am comfortable with my knowledge and skills it is easier to practice the art of being fully present, without the anxiety that comes with feeling unprepared, and lacking in expertise and knowledge.

This workbook is specifically written for nursing students, and nurses interested in a self study guide. It is also intended as a resource for nursing instructors. If you are using this as part of a "class" you may have sections assigned to complete, participate in small group discussion/role plays etc. If using this as a self study guide I encourage you to use it in whatever way helps you to reflect on your own beliefs, interact with the concepts and content, and apply theory in practice. You may want to request input from a mentor, gather a group to facilitate learning, and/or request clinical supervision to assist in implementation.

I invite you to send me feedback on what was helpful, not helpful, and any suggestions for improvement. I am also happy to collect your stories!

I express gratitude for Elizabeth Causton and Terry Downing who contributed to the development, and to Ann-Marie Gilbert who continues to provide great editorial support.

I dedicate this workbook to Krystal (Murray) Brown a Licensed Practical Nurse who also happens to be my daughter.

Contents

Instructions for Workbook Activities

This workbook includes activities designed to assist learners to understand and integrate the concepts and content into their practice.

Reflective Writing

In the section "Beliefs and Baggage" learners are asked to write "reflectively." This is a style of writing wherein authors write down all thoughts and ideas in response to a statement, question or comment. It is important in reflective writing to allow all thoughts to be written and to resist censuring or editing your own writing. This enables the writer to "hear" their own thoughts and express them in writing. The process of reflective writing is shown to assist individuals in understanding their own ideas, beliefs and potential biases about each topic and may help them to connect with new theory by bringing a greater understanding of themselves to the topic.

Short and Long Answer Questions

Writing exercises include definitions as well as short and long answer questions. These exercises emphasize the basic concepts and content of each topic and will provide the foundation for Integration and Application work.

Group Discussions

Group activities are the primary learning tools in Integration and Application. There are three types of group activities in this workbook - small group discussions, large group discussions and role playing.

Small group discussions are designed to focus your attention on the details of discussion with your colleagues and to work collectively in determining how to apply concepts and to enhance your understanding.

Large group discussions are either follow up sessions with the larger group or after completing your own reading and research. Working with many individuals enables you to check in with your own learning and to develop a broader base of understanding of concepts. In the group discussions you will see how cases are viewed differently, based on different context, different people and different family. You will see how the interventions will differ based on who is involved.

Case Studies

Case studies provide an opportunity to apply new knowledge and skills. Refer to these questions for consideration at the beginning of each case study.

- What is the meaning of this symptom to the patient?
- How does this symptom affects the patient's lifestyle?
- How does the patient rate this symptom as compared to other symptoms they are experiencing?
- What are the patient's priorities in symptom management?

Role Plays

Role plays are essential to learning caregiving skills. In the same manner that we practice the physical aspects of caregiving to develop the muscle memory of the activity, we also benefit from practicing the communication skills for caregiving to develop the psychological memory of a practice experience. This will enhance your capacity to communicate effectively with patients and family as they deal with the complex emotional issues of dying. In role plays, assume each of these three different roles with the following expectations:

- Observer - As observer your role is to "watch" and identify what went well, what the caregiver may have added, missed or left out.

- Caregiver - As caregiver you will be expected to integrate the materials from the manual and use the given tools to assess, document and report. If you need input from the observer and the patient, it is appropriate to ask for this support.

- Patient - As a patient you will be expected to "fill in the blanks" to "add the life story" and to identify the pieces that make each patient unique.

Answers

Answer for the workbook can be accessed at www.lifeanddeathmatters.ca in the Learning Centre.

Introduction to Hospice Palliative Care

Beliefs and Baggage

1. One piece of baggage that we all carry involves our own biases about what constitutes a 'good' or 'bad' death for ourselves. Write your own list of the characteristics of a 'good' and 'bad' death. _____

_____

_____

_____

2. Write about the origins of your beliefs about a 'good/bad' death e.g family, culture, religion, workplace, personal experience. _____

_____

_____

_____

_____

_____

3. List and explore the similarities and differences between the lists of 'good' and 'bad' deaths compiled by you and your class mates. _____

_____

_____

_____

_____

4. Contraction Exercise

In the large box on the next page, write the things that are important for you to do in your life.

In the medium circle, write the things that might be important for you to do if you only had three months to live.

In the center circle, write the things that you would want to do if you only had three days left to live.

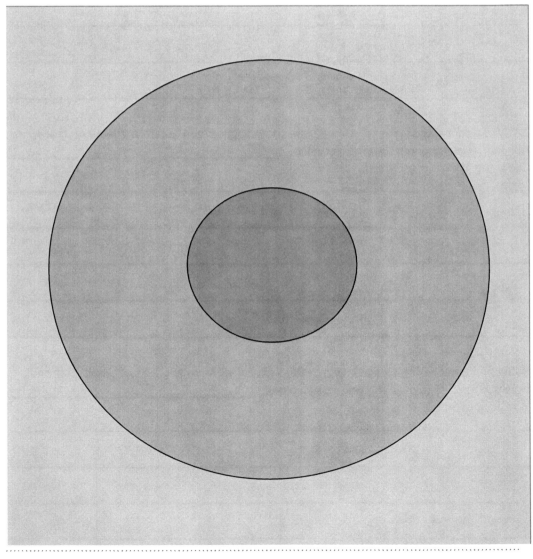

5. How might you feel if you did not get to decide what you could do with your
remaining days because someone had decided for you? _____

_____

_____

_____

_____

_____

Concepts and Content

Definitions

6. Palliative_____

_____

_____

7. Hospice _____

_____

_____

8. End of life care _____

_____

_____

9. Appropriate death_____

_____

_____

10. Ambiguous dying syndrome _____

_____

_____

11. Do you have a Palliative Care Benefits program in your province? What are the criteria for registration? (For more information go to www.health.gov.bc.ca/pharme/outgoing/palliative.html)._____

_____

_____

12. The Compassionate Caregivers program is offered by the Canadian Government. How does a family member access this resource? (www.compassionatecaregivers.ca/caregivers.html)._____

_____

_____

Integration and Application

Small or Large Group Discussions

13. Compare the definition of your 'good/bad' death to the definition of an 'appropriate death.' What challenges might you encounter in facilitating an appropriate death for an individual whose "good/bad" death list is different from yours? _____

_____

_____

_____

_____

_____

14. What are three questions that you could ask that would enable you to better understand the patient's and family's perspective on what would be a 'good/bad' death? Compare this list in small group discussion and expand the list. _____

_____

_____

_____

_____

_____

_____

15. Choose three ways to facilitate an appropriate death from the list on page 17 of Essentials, and describe how you would implement them in the context of your role as a caregiver. _____

_____

_____

_____

_____

_____

_____

_____

_____

16. Allowing family to be involved to whatever extent they wish is a principle of HPC. How do you support a family member who DOES NOT want to be involved in the caregiving process? How do you support family who DOES want to be very involved?

These questions may be answered by dividing into two groups, each discussing one question. When finished the groups can come together to discuss.

_____

_____

_____

_____

_____

_____

_____

_____

_____

_____

_____

_____

_____

_____

_____

Enhancing Comfort and Managing Symptoms

Introduction and Tools
Beliefs and Baggage

1. Describe your beliefs about physical comfort. What does this term mean to you? _____

_____

_____

_____

2. Explore the roles of different members of the care team in contributing to an assessment. Why do you feel that each of these different perspectives is important?_____

_____

_____

_____

_____

_____

3. Describe what you would appreciate being asked if someone was assessing your pain.

_____

_____

_____

_____

Content and Concepts

CHPCA Process of Providing Care

Short Answer Questions

4. Two components of the CHPCA Process of Providing Care that are not traditionally identified in the caregiving process are *Sharing Information* and *Decision Making*. Give examples of open ended questions that might help you identify how to best share information with patients and families.

> *Example: "How do you like to receive information? Alone? In a family meeting?"*

_____

_____

_____

_____

_____

_____

5. Describe what appropriate information sharing with the patient and family would look like, given your role on the health care team. Give two examples. _____

_____

_____

_____

_____

_____

_____

_____

6. Describe two ways that you might facilitate information sharing from the health care team to the patient and family, given the family's preferences. _____

_____

_____

_____

_____

_____

7. Based on the common issues as described by the CHPCA Square of Care, what are three decisions that families might struggle with at end of life? (See Essentials manual, page 23)

Example: How to manage symptoms.

_____

_____

_____

_____

_____

8. Considering the diversity of the common issues, identify diverse members of the health care team who may be involved in the care of this patient/family. Explain the referral process._____

_____

_____

_____

_____

Common Issues

Short Answer Questions and Small Group Discussions

9. List eight common issues identified in the Square of Care. _____

_____

_____

_____

_____

10. Identify three things you might assess within each of 3 issues. _____

_____

_____

_____

_____

Tools

11. Describe the value of using standardized tools for assessments. _____

_____

_____

_____

_____

12. Describe the purpose of the Palliative Performance Scale (PPS). _____

_____

_____

13. Go online to read the guidelines for using the Edmonton Symptom Assessment Acronym (ESAS). Describe 4 guidelines for using the ESAS correctly.

_____

_____

_____

_____

14. What will the ESAS tool help you to identify? (Essentials, pg 29). _____

_____

15. Describe the meaning of the letters *OPQRSTUV* in the Fraser Health Symptom Assessment Acronym (FHSAA). List sample questions to ask for each of the letters.

_____

_____

_____

_____

_____

_____

_____

16. Where would you find the guidelines for using the FHSAA? List guidelines for using the FHSAA correctly. _____

_____

_____

_____

_____

_____

_____

_____

_____

17. Read the section on "Explorer versus Detective" in Essentials, pg 26-27. Explain the difference in the focus of these approaches in your own words. _____

_____

_____

_____

_____

_____

_____

_____

18. What do the letters *SBAR* represent? How might this communication tool be useful for you in your practice? _____

_____

_____

_____

_____

_____

_____

Principles for Using Medication to Manage Symptoms

19. Describe at least six principles in using medications to manage symptoms. _____

_____

_____

_____

_____

_____

_____

_____

_____

_____

_____

20. List a minimum of 5 common symptoms experienced by the dying.

_____

_____

_____

_____

_____

_____

_____

_____

_____

_____

Integration and Application

Small Group Discussions

21. Together with your colleagues, develop a list of 25 things you might do to offer comfort, e.g. physical support, resources and psychosocial support. _____

_____

_____

_____

_____

_____

_____

_____

_____

_____

_____

_____

22. Discuss when to assess a patient for comfort. _____

_____

_____

_____

_____

Using Tools in Assessments

Large Group Discussions

23. Prepare answers for large group discussions. Use the space below for notes.

- Discuss the commonalities in the uses of the tools ESAS, PAIN AD and the FHSAA. What are the features that make each a unique assessment tool?
- What are the differences between questions that elicit facts, ie. *OPQRST,* and those that help us understand the story of what pain means for this person, i.e. *UV?*
- Describe how assessments of individuals with dementia are different from those of individuals with normal mentation.
- What is different when assessing someone who is non-responsive?
- Discuss the importance of involving the family/significant others in client care.

_____

_____

_____

_____

_____

_____

_____

_____

_____

_____

_____

_____

24. Keeping in mind the diagram of the health care team, (Essentials, pg 19) who on the team is involved with assessing patient comfort and symptoms? _____

_____

_____

_____

_____

25. While keeping the values of using standardized tools for assessments in mind, what might the challenges be in acknowledging each patient's unique experience or context?

_____

_____

_____

Using Tools to Document and Communicate Assessments to Physicians

26. You want to do an initial assessment of a patient on admission. List the benefits of using the ESAS in general and specifically for Case Study #3 (see Essentials, pg 30) then discuss your findings with a colleague. _____

_____

_____

_____

_____

_____

_____

_____

27. Discuss the guidelines for using the ESAS correctly with the larger group. _____

_____

_____

_____

_____

_____

_____

_____

28. Would the FHSAA be useful for Case Study #3? Discuss why or why not. _____

_____

_____

_____

_____

_____

_____

_____

Large Group Demonstrations

29. Observe a demonstration on positioning patients in bed for comfort, using pillows, stuffies, and blankets. In small groups, implement the strategy and discuss how best to work with patients when positioning for comfort. Use blank space on next page for notes.

30. Watch a demonstration of hand massage. Perform and/or teach hand massage to another individual. Use the blank portion of this page for notes.

Role Play and Large Group Discussion

31. Using role play, demonstrate first a "bad pain assessment" and then a "good pain assessment." When completed, discuss in the group the characteristics of each assessment. _____

_____

_____

_____

_____

_____

Pain
Beliefs and Baggage

1. Reflect on a time when you had a tooth ache. Describe that pain._____

_____

_____

_____

2. Reflect on a time when you experienced a sun burn, shingles, or a cold sore. Describe that pain._____

_____

_____

_____

3. Reflect on a time when you had kidney stones, were experiencing labour pains associated with delivery or were constipated. Describe that pain. _____

_____

_____

_____

4. What are your beliefs about the use of medications to control pain? _____

_____

_____

_____

_____

5. Identify two of your favorite comfort measures to receive. _____

_____

_____

6. Identify two comfort measures that you offer as part of your daily care._____

_____

_____

Concepts and Content

Definitions

7. Pain _____

_____

8. Total pain _____

_____

9. "Pain" according to the "Association for Pain." _____

_____

_____

10. "Pain" according to Margot McCaffery. _____

_____

11. Identify times when McCaffery's definition of pain may not be helpful.

_____

_____

12. Nociceptive pain _____

_____

_____

13. List examples of nociceptive, visceral, and somatic pain. _____

_____

_____

_____

_____

14. Neuropathic pain _____

_____

_____

15. List 3 examples of neuropathic pain. _____

_____

16. Palliation _____

_____

17. Titrate/titration _____

_____

_____

18. Breakthrough doses _____

_____

19. What other words might be used to refer to the breakthrough dose? _____

_____

20. Adjuvant medications _____

_____

21. What are 3 non-pharmacological comfort measures? _____

_____

_____

Short Answer Questions

22. List five adjuvant medications used in pain management and briefly explain how they contribute to pain management. _____

_____

_____

_____

_____

_____

23. Explain ten principles of pain management (Essentials, pg 44). _____

_____

_____

_____

_____

_____

_____

_____

_____

_____

_____

_____

_____

_____

_____

_____

_____

Integration and Application

Role Play

24. Use a role play to determine the symptoms Robert is facing. Prepare to discuss your findings with the larger group. Use the space below for notes.

_____

_____

_____

_____

_____

_____

_____

_____

_____

_____

_____

25. Consider and discuss the following questions.

      a. When should pain be assessed?
      b. Who assesses pain?
      c. What non-verbal behaviours may indicate pain?
      d. Discuss different types of pain.
      e. Identify comfort measures that may support someone in pain.

_____

_____

_____

_____

_____

_____

_____

_____

_____

_____

_____

_____

_____

_____

Using Opioids to Manage Pain
Content and Concepts

Short Answer Questions

1. If it is not the responsibility of the RN or the LPN to order pain medications then why is the information on equianalgesia and titration included in this workbook? Why is it helpful to understand the equianalgesia chart, the different methods of titration and other information about opioids? _____

_____

_____

_____

_____

2. List four common side effects of using opioids. _____

_____

_____

_____

3. Explain four common myths about opioids. _____

_____

_____

_____

Note: Allergic responses to opioids are very rare. If a hypersensitivity reaction - including rash, wheezing and edema occur then contact the physician. It may be necessary to switch to a different or a synthetic opioid.

4. List 4 comfort measures to prevent constipation in the dying. _____

_____

_____

_____

_____

Opioid Orders

Calculations with Short Answers

5. Identify problems with the analgesic orders as written.

a. Morphine 10-15 mg *p.o. q4-6h prn* for severe pain._____

_____

_____

b. Tylenol #3 1-2 *p.o. q6h prn* mild-moderate pain. _____

_____

_____

c. Morphine 20 mg *p.o. q4h* and morphine 5 mg for breakthrough dose (BTD) as needed. _____

_____

_____

d. Fentanyl patch 25 mcg *q72h.* _____

_____

_____

6. Describe why opioids are given regularly, (i.e. every four hours) around the clock.

_____

_____

_____

_____

_____

Exercises in Equianalgesia for Opioids

Equianalgesia Table for Opioids

Drug	Oral/ Rectal	Sub-cutaneous	Schedule
		Route	
codeine	100mg	65mg	q4h
oxycodone	5.0 to 7.0 mg	-	q4h
morphine	10 mg	5 mg	q4h
hydromorphone (Dilaudid®)	2 mg	1 mg	q4h
fentanyl patch (Duragesic®)	25 ug/hr patch = 60 to 134 mg total oral daily dose of morphine	-	q72h

Note: It is not the role of the nurse to determine the exact dosage of opioid in conversions. Instead, the nurses role is to be famaliar with the calculations and aware of appropriate dose ranges so that they will be able to help identify when a mistake is made in conversion, or to identify when the opioid order needs to be adjusted to better meet the needs of the patient.

Complete the following calculations.

7. A patient is currently taking Tylenol #3 - 2 tabs *qid* (Each Tylenol #3 contains 325 mg of acetaminophen and 30 mg codeine).

a. Calculate this patient's 24 hour dose of codeine. _____

_____

_____

b. Calculate this patient's 4 hour dose of codeine. _____

_____

_____

c. Calculate the equianalgesia dose of the following medications for this patient:

    i. Morphine oral *q4h* _____

    ii. Morphine Contin *q12h* _____

    iii. Morphine subcutaneous _____

8. A patient is currently taking Morphine 30mg *p.o. q4h*, and the physician has ordered a switch to Dilaudid.

  a. Dilaudid oral *q4h* _____

  b. Hydromorph Contin *p.o. q12h* _____

  c. Dilaudid *s.c. q4h* _____

  d. Transderm Fentanyl (see note below) _____

> **Conversion for Fentanyl Patch:** When switching to Fentanyl Patch, the wide range of doses makes it difficult to complete the calculation. Therefore, for the purpose of the exercises pertaining to Fentanyl in this book please use the following conversion:
> Fentanyl 25ug/hour = Morphine 96 mg/24hours.

Calculating Breakthrough Doses

9. What are the formulas for determining breakthrough doses? _____

_____

_____

10. What formula is used in the area where you work? _____

_____

11 A physician is ordering Dilaudid 10 mg *s.c. q4h*. What would be an appropriate breakthrough dose? Why? _____

_____

_____

12. The physician has ordered Morphine 50 mg *p.o. q4h* and Morphine 5 mg *p.o.* for a breakthrough dose.

a. What is the problem with the breakthrough dose? Why? _____

_____

_____

b. What formula did you use for determining breakthrough doses?_____

_____

c. What is an appropriate breakthrough dose? _____

_____

_____

13. Calculate the appropriate breakthrough dose for a patient receiving Morphine Contin 60 mg *p.o. q12h*? _____

_____

_____

14. What medication can be used as a breakthrough dose for a patient receiving Fentanyl 25 mcg/hour patch and why? What should the breakthrough dose be?_____

_____

_____

Opioid Titration

Calculations

Case Study #2

Daniel Hyghbroughten, a patient, rates his pain at a 6/10. The current dose of morphine is 30 mg *p.o. q4h* (180 mg/day). However Daniel took 4 breakthrough doses (15 mg *p.o.* Morphine) in past 24 hours.

Calculate new opioid doses for these cases using the three methods listed.

15 a. *Method #1*, Increase dose by amount of the interim dose _____

_____

_____

b. *Method #2*, Increase according to total daily dose _____

_____

_____

c. *Method #3*, Increase by percentage _____

_____

Case Study #3

Lance Fjeldstad, rates his pain at 4/10. No BTDs were used in past 24 hours. Current dose of Dilaudid is 10 mg *s.c. q4h*, BTD 5 mg *s.c. prn*. Family is finding it difficult to make decisions about giving extra pain medications. Lance wants the pain settled to at least 1/10. He is currently unable to sleep because of waking with pain.

16 a. *Method* #1, Increase by amount of the interim dose _____

_____

_____

b. *Method* #2, Increase according to total daily dose _____

_____

_____

c. *Method* #3, Increase by percentage _____

_____

_____

Integration and Application

Small Group Discussions

17. Compare the calculated opioid doses and discuss reasons for dosage differences when using Method #1 in Case Study #1 and Case Study #2. _____

_____

_____

_____

_____

_____

_____

_____

Side Effects, Fears and Myths of Using Opioids

Case Study #4

Upon return to work after days off you are again assigned to Robert, the 65 years old, male, with cancer of prostate and a recent diagnosis of metastases/spread to bone. We rejoin him on his third day on the unit when he was very slow getting out of bed. He holds his right hip, supports himself by holding on to furniture as he moves. This is very different from the past two days. Initially he denies pain, though admits to being "sore". You complete a pain assessment with Robert.

In discussing his pain, Robert rates his pain at 5/10. This is the same pain location from before however it is increasing. You review his current pain medications which no longer control the pain.

Robert is currently taking morphine 5 mg p.o. q4h. He has orders for breakthrough medication if he experiences any pain, but is reluctant to take any.

You explore with him his concerns about using opioids and realize that he is concerned about taking any opioid at all! Robert vehemently states,

"I do not like taking morphine at all.... and I am worried about getting constipated, and other side effects, and about being addicted... you know...to the medicine."

Small Group Discussions

18. Discuss the side effects of opioids and why Robert might be concerned about them.

_____

_____

_____

_____

_____

19. Discuss in small groups how to respond to his concerns, considering your role on the health care team. _____

_____

_____

20. Robert states that his family is very concerned about his being on morphine EVERY four hours(!) Discuss in small groups how to teach family about the need for medication every four hours. Use diagrams to support your discussion. _____

_____

_____

_____

_____

Robert states that the family believes that if he is taking morphine, it means that he is going to die?

21. Considering your role on the health care team, how might you respond to this concern? _____

_____

_____

_____

_____

22. Identify opioid uses, side effects, fears, and teaching regarding use of opioids around the clock (RTC). _____

_____

_____

_____

_____

Titrating with Opioids

Case Study #5

You come on shift and get the following report:

Brenda Selkirk, a 55 y/o woman with metastatic breast cancer was admitted to your unit last night, via emergency. She has severe back pain. Rates it at 6-8/10. Brenda is unable to walk or sit due to the pain that has become worse over the past weeks.

Medication review: At home Brenda was taking Dilaudid 2 mg *p.o. q4h*, with little effect. She did not take any BTDs.

Brenda was seen by the emergency room physician, during a very busy shift in emergency. The following orders were written: Dilaudid 2 mg *p.o. q4-6h* prn severe pain. Oncologist consult requested to see if radiation can be done to decrease pain.

The next morning (11 hours after admission) report indicates that Brenda is still in pain. You review the chart. No thorough pain assessment has been completed. From the chart it is unclear where the pain is located and any other information about the pain. Cancer clinic records are not available. Medication records reveal that she only received Dilaudid 2 mg at 2200 and 0400.

Role Play

23. Assess, document and communicate Brenda's pain assessment using the Fraser Health Symptom Assessment Acronym. _____

_____

_____

_____

_____

24. What is Brenda's goal for pain management? _____

_____

_____

_____

25. Use the SBAR and write your communication with the physician about the patient's pain. _____

_____

_____

_____

26. Describe problems with the opioid orders given in the E.R. _____

_____

_____

_____

_____

26. Why do some physicians order *prn* for ongoing pain? _____

_____

_____

_____

Titration of Medications

Case Study #6

Brenda is very anxious to have pain controlled NOW!

You suggest to the physician a route change to *s.c.* until pain is settled, a new dose determined and she is able to return to *p.o.* medications. Calculate the doses for sample route changes Use Equianalgesia Table for assistance.

27. Using Method #1, Method #2, or Method #3, identify what dose you might use? Show calculations. _____

_____

_____

_____

_____

_____

_____

_____

Assessing Pain with Dementia
Integration and Application

Case Study #7

Sarah Mussell is an 89 year old female with osteoarthritis, breast cancer, a fractured hip and Alzheimer's dementia in her history. Today, Sarah calls out and hits you when you attempt to give morning care and transfer. You discuss her needs and review her chart with team mates.

- Sarah is not able to communicate verbally using words.
- Her condition has been declining over the past months.
- She has refused solids for the past week but has taken fluids with encouragement.
- In particular, Sarah shows decreased mobility and resists getting transferred out of bed.
- She has become increasingly withdrawn, no longer engaging with music therapist.
- Sarah has had four infections in past six months with a poor response to antibiotics.

Medications: Tylenol 2 tabs *tid* for past month. According to chart this appeared to assist with comfort during transfers.

Family is concerned that she is in pain. No recent pain assessment on chart.

Small and Large Group Discussions, Role Play

28. Discuss and role play in small groups to answer these questions about the case study. Prepare your findings to share in the large group discussion. Use the next page for notes.
    - Who are you going to consult with as you assess her pain?
    - What tools can you use to assess her pain?
    - Discuss and compare the uses of ESAS, Symptom Assessment Acronym, and PAIN AD.
        - Which tools would be helpful?
        - Discuss the pros and cons of using these tools.
        - Will the PAINAD identify the presence of pain or provide you with the severity of pain?
    - Discuss the unique aspects of assessing pain with someone with dementia.

Role play,

Assess Sarah's pain, document the findings, and use the SBAR to communicate your findings. _____

_____

_____

_____

_____

_____

_____

_____

_____

_____

_____

_____

_____

_____

_____

_____

_____

Dyspnea

Beliefs and Baggage

1. With your colleagues, complete the exercise on breathing through a straw on page 61 of Essentials and write about your experience. Following the exercise, take some slow deep breaths to help restore comfortable breathing.

_____

_____

_____

_____

_____

_____

_____

_____

_____

_____

_____

_____

_____

2. What are your personal experiences with difficult breathing? Describe how this exercise has changed your perception of being short of breath. _____

_____

_____

_____

_____

_____

_____

_____

3. What words did your colleagues use to describe their experience of being short of breath? How do their words compare to yours? What does this tell you about the subjectiveness of the experience of shortness of breath? _____

_____

_____

_____

_____

_____

_____

Concepts and Content

Definitions and Short Answer Questions

4. Define dyspnea _____

_____

_____

_____

5. Does the experience of dyspnea always relate to the oxygen saturation level? _____

_____

_____

_____

6. Do patients always report their dyspnea? _____

_____

_____

7. What words/phrases might trigger you to assess dyspnea? _____

_____

_____

8. Why are opioids helpful in relieving dyspnea? _____

_____

_____

_____

9. Identify comfort measures for dyspnea. _____

_____

_____

_____

10. Describe four key points in managing dyspnea. _____

_____

_____

_____

_____

Note: You may want to refer to the Refer to the Registered Nurses Association of Ontario, online for "best practice" documents on dyspnea.

Integration and Application

Assessing Dyspnea

Case Study #8

Jason Maher, 52 years old, with cancer of the esophagus that has spread to the liver. On arrival you notice that Jason is very short of breath (SOB). He acknowledges that he is SOB, it is quite uncomfortable, rates discomfort at 7/10. He appears anxious but does not like to complain.

Role Play

11. In role play, develop and give the SBAR summary of the dyspnea assessment to a physician. When preparing the report for the physician, include in your assessment:

• Ativan has not been effective.

- Bronchodilators have not worked.
- He has no need of diuretics.

_____

_____

_____

_____

12. Using the Symptom Assessment Acronym and referring to the Fraser Health website, (Fraser Health Symptom Control Guidelines, www.fraserhealth.ca) what questions would you ask to assess Jason's dyspnea?_____

_____

_____

_____

_____

13. As an explorer, what questions might help you to identify the patient's subjective experience of dyspnea, in terms of understanding and value?_____

_____

_____

_____

_____

14. List physical behaviours that you might observe with dyspnea which would be helpful in completing your assessment._____

_____

_____

15. Record your assessment of Jason's breathing. _____

_____

_____

_____

_____

16. Jason asks you what the word "dyspnea" means. Describe two different ways to explain this concept to your patient. _____

_____

_____

_____

_____

_____

Managing Dyspnea

17. What is the role of "calmness" in responding to dyspnea? _____

_____

_____

_____

_____

18. Using role play (either in a large group or in pairs) coach a person who is role playing being short of breath. Follow suggestions in the manual and debrief as a class.

19. In role play, integrate comfort strategies that you can offer to a patient experiencing dyspnea. _____

_____

_____

_____

_____

_____

Large Group Discussions

20. What palliative measures can you offer to manage dyspnea?_____

_____

_____

_____

21. Identify the principles for using opioids to manage dyspnea._____

_____

_____

_____

_____

_____

22. Describe the process for titrating opioids for a person with dyspnea. How is this similar or different than if the person were in pain? _____

_____

_____

_____

23. Using the Fraser Health symptom management guidelines, describe other medications (besides opioids) that could be useful with dyspnea. Include any additional information you would need to determine whether other medications would be useful._

_____

_____

_____

24. Give an example of a sedative that might be useful. _____

_____

25. Develop a resource list of current, local, best practice websites and articles on dyspnea to use as a resource to share with physicians. _____

_____

_____

_____

_____

_____

_____

_____

Case Study #9

Barbara Caldwell is 79 years with end stage cardiac disease and COPD.

History - sudden difficulty breathing at night, and ongoing shortness of breath (SOB) with activity. SOB increases with movement in past month, today particularly difficult following eating, and when she talks (often pauses when speaking). Mobility limited to transfer to commode. Difficulty rating dyspnea but suggests 6/10. Fatigue and feeling of weakness over past weeks has been increasing. Pulse oximetry was not taken.

Observations – Edema: +3 legs up to knees. Uses auxiliary muscles for breathing when SOB. Gasps when SOB. Resp rate 30/min, pulse 100 per minute. Less alert. Periods of confusion in past few days. Skin cool, clammy, diaphoretic. Changing condition, no solids for 24 hours *NPO*, mouth care only today.

26. Discuss comfort measures that might be helpful to implement right away._____

_____

_____

_____

_____

27. When the family asks "Would oxygen would be helpful?", how would you reply? What information do you need to answer this questions? _____

_____

_____

_____

_____

28. The family asks if suctioning secretions in her mouth would be helpful. What is your response? Explain your answer. _____

_____

_____

_____

_____

_____

_____

29. Which medications could be helpful for Barbara and why? _____

_____

_____

_____

30. Describe the principles for using opioids in managing dyspnea. _____

_____

_____

_____

_____

_____

31. Could Barbara be dying? Explain your answer._____

_____

_____

_____

32. Read page 113 to 115 of Essentials on dying with chronic illness. Referring to the case study of Barbara, what are the challenges for prognosticating for people with chronic illness? (She has been very sick before and she got better.) _____

_____

_____

_____

_____

_____

_____

_____

Demonstration

Teaching a person to clear the secretions in their chest

Using the information at the website for registered nurses of Ontario, download and print the best practice guidelines for persons with COPD, at http://www.rnao.org/ Storage/11/604_BPG_COPD.pdf, Appendix H.

Small Group Discussion

33. How you would integrate this information into your practice? _____

_____

_____

_____

_____

_____

_____

_____

_____

_____

_____

_____

_____

Note: As death becomes more imminent a person will be unable to do this exercise.

Pre-death Respiratory Congestion
Beliefs and Baggage

1. Write about your associations with the term "death rattle" in terms of physical comfort. _____

_____

_____

_____

_____

_____

_____

_____

2. What are your beliefs about pre-death respiratory congestion in the context of a 'good/bad' death? _____

_____

_____

_____

_____

_____

_____

_____

3. Discuss, in pairs, your beliefs about a patient's awareness of symptoms such as respiratory congestion as they near death. What is this belief based on? _____

_____

_____

_____

Concepts and Content

Short Answer Questions

4. Describe causes of pre-death respiratory congestion. _____

_____

_____

_____

_____

5. List common medications used to control respiratory congestion._____

_____

_____

_____

_____

6. Describe comfort measures for respiratory congestion. _____

_____

_____

_____

7. Explain the information families might find useful regarding pre-death respiratory congestion. _____

_____

_____

_____

Integration and Application

8. Explain how you would assess respiratory congestion as the patient nears death and how to determine the patient's comfort level? _____

_____

_____

_____

_____

Large Group Discussion

9. In the large group, discuss ways to enhance the patient's physical comfort while also managing the family's concerns. _____

_____

_____

_____

_____

_____

_____

_____

Nausea and Vomiting
Beliefs and Baggage

1. From your own personal experience, describe your beliefs about nausea and vomiting (N/V). _____

_____

_____

_____

_____

_____

_____

_____

2. List comfort measures that you find helpful and those that you do not find helpful when you are vomiting. _____

_____

_____

_____

_____

_____

Concepts and Content

3. Identify and label at least ten causes of nausea/vomiting on the body map below. Use the Fraser Health website and Essentials manual for references.

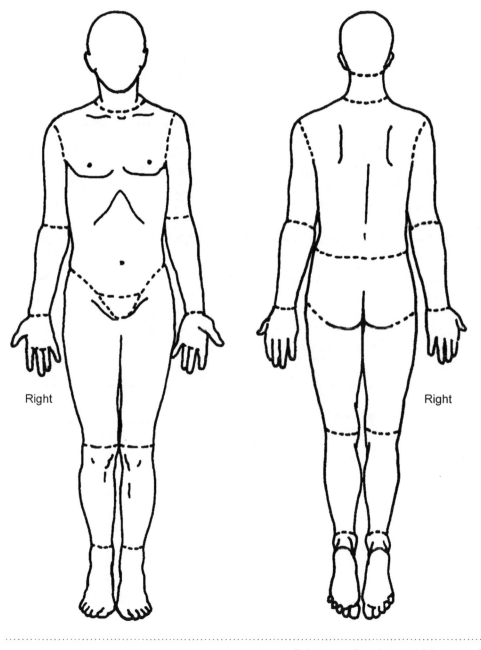

Right

Right

4. In this list below, link the cause of nausea with one of the most appropriate medications to help decrease the nausea and vomiting.

Haldol or Nozinan   bowel obstruction caused by tumour pressing on intestines

Gravol   constipation

Dexamethasone   vomiting partially digested food

Maxeran   started on opioid and immediately vomited

Sennokot   motion sickness

5. List and explain key points in using medications to manage N/V. _____

_____

_____

_____

_____

6. Describe comfort strategies for N/V. _____

_____

_____

_____

_____

7. Draw on personal, clinical and theoretical experiences as well as the acronym *OPQRSTUV* to create questions to assess a person's nausea and vomiting. _____

_____

_____

_____

_____

_____

_____

_____

_____

_____

_____

_____

_____

_____

_____

_____

_____

_____

_____

Integration and Application

Small Group Discussion

8. Compile a list of questions based on the *OPQRSTUV* to assess the causes, severity, and frequency of nausea and vomiting. Remember to explore the patient's priorities in symptom management._____

_____

_____

_____

_____

_____

Large Group Discussions

9. Explain why different types of medications may be needed to palliate nausea and vomiting resulting from different causes. _____

_____

_____

_____

_____

_____

_____

_____

10. Discuss the principles for using medications for palliation as described on page 75 and 76, Essentials. _____

_____

_____

_____

_____

_____

_____

Cachexia and Anorexia
Beliefs and Baggage

1. Imagine that you look in the mirror and you have lost so much weight that you do not recognize the person who stares back at you. Reflect and write about your feelings._____

_____

_____

_____

2. Describe how the following two scenarios might be different:

"You have the flu and you are nauseated" versus "You are sick with cancer and you are nauseated"

_____

_____

_____

_____

3. Reflect on the role of food in nurturing in your family. Hypothesize and describe reasons why a decreasing appetite could be a difficult symptom for your family to witness._____

_____

_____

_____

_____

_____

4. Identify five "Food for Thought" points about decreasing intake that resonate for you.

_____

_____

_____

_____

Concepts and Content

Definitions and Short Answer Questions

5. Define anorexia _____

_____

_____

6. Define cachexia _____

_____

_____

7. List and/or explain information about anorexia and cachexia that might be helpful for families. _____

_____

_____

_____

_____

_____

_____

Integration and Application

8. Prepare a comparison of appropriate nourishment for a person whose age is: 1 day, 1 month, 1 year, 10 years, 20 years, 40 years, 60 years, 80 years and 100 years? Describe or depict this in a diagram.

9. Describe what would happen if you gave the food eaten by the 20 year old to the 80 year old, a) 1 time, b) on a regular basis, and c) at bedtime. _____

_____

_____

_____

_____

_____

_____

10. Describe what would happen if you gave only food for a 1 year old to the 20 year old on a regular basis. _____

_____

_____

_____

_____

11. How do these questions help to understand the term "appropriate nourishment" for the dying? _____

_____

_____

_____

12. Discuss whether "Food for Thought" helps you understand the decreased need for intake when a person is dying. Why or why not?_____

_____

_____

_____

_____

_____

_____

Large Group Discussion

Dr. Edwardo Bruera teaches, "Tell your dying patients and their families that the stomach is on strike"

13. What is helpful about this particular statement?_____

_____

_____

14. Discuss your role to assess, advocate and educate. _____

_____

_____

_____

_____

_____

_____

Role Play

Use Role play, portray a nurse discussing concerns about decreasing intake with a family member. From Sarah's previous case history, we know that she has

- Shown declining health over past months,
- Refused solids for the past week. Taken fluids with encouragement,
- In particular shown decreased mobility, resists getting transferred out of bed,
- Become increasingly withdrawn, no longer engaging with music therapist,
- Shown poor response to antibiotic treatment for four infections in past six months,
- Medication changed to Tylenol 2 tabs tid for past month. According to chart this appeared to assist with comfort during transfers.

15. What words might you use to explain the decreased need for food, and decreased ability to tolerate food? _____

_____

_____

_____

16. Debrief this topic with the large group.

Oral Discomfort
Beliefs and Baggage

1. Describe your experiences with sores in the mouth. _____

_____

_____

2. What aspects of daily living are affected by having oral discomfort? _____

_____

_____

3. Give three reasons why oral discomfort might be missed in the assessment process.___

_____

_____

_____

Concepts and Content

4. List common causes of oral discomfort. _____

_____

_____

_____

5. Why is thrush a common infection in the dying? _____

_____

_____

6. What does thrush look like? _____

_____

_____

Integration and Application

7. Describe what you would assess when a patient has a sore mouth. _____

_____

_____

_____

8. What comfort strategies can you implement? How would these strategies differ for different causes of discomfort? _____

_____

_____

_____

Dehydration
Beliefs and Baggage

1. Describe a personal experience with being dehydrated. What did you do about it? ____

_____

_____

_____

_____

_____

2. What are your beliefs about the need for hydration through to death? Are there any exceptions? _____

_____

_____

_____

_____

3. What are the origins of these beliefs? _____

_____

_____

_____

_____

Concepts and Content

Large Group Discussions

4. Describe why dehydration is a normal part of dying for many people._____

_____

_____

_____

_____

5. Explain why dehydration is treated in some cases and is considered inappropriate to treat in other cases._____

_____

_____

_____

6. Identify three possible disadvantages of dehydration in the last days and hours of a person's life. _____

_____

_____

7. Identify three possible benefits of dehydration in the last days and hours of a person's life._____

_____

_____

_____

Integration and Application

A family member is asking questions about why their loved one is not receiving hydration.

> "I know they are dying in a few days but they aren't drinking or eating anything – will they be uncomfortable?"

Role Play

8. Use a role play to :

- Determine the family's beliefs about the appropriateness of dehydration as death nears.
- Assess the family's observations and impressions of the patient's level of comfort.
- Explore the family's own experiences and understanding of dehydration.

_____

_____

_____

_____

Large Group Discussion

9. Integrating information from the previous role play, discuss ways to explain the advantages and disadvantages of dehydration with dying to family. _____

_____

_____

_____

_____

_____

10. Describe ways the family can continue to comfort and nurture the patient without involving artificial hydration. _____

_____

_____

_____

_____

_____

_____

_____

_____

_____

Delirium
Beliefs and Baggage

1. What are your beliefs and associations with the symptom of delirium? _____

_____

_____

_____

2. Compare and describe your impressions of using the word "delirium" as compared to "confusion". How do you think family members would respond to each of these terms?

_____

_____

3. Why might delirium be frightening to patients or family? _____

_____

_____

_____

Concepts and Content

Short Answer Questions

4. Describe different causes of delirium._____

_____

_____

_____

_____

5. Which of these causes are normal changes in the dying process? _____

_____

_____

_____

6. What are five characteristics of delirium? Essentials, pgs 93 to 94._____

_____

_____

_____

_____

_____

7. When would treating delirium be questionable? _____

_____

_____

_____

Integration and Application

8. How would the FHSAA be helpful? Is it appropriate to ask Allan what he remembers about his confusion in the night? _____

_____

_____

_____

_____

_____

9. What questions might you ask about goals of care and investigations?_____

_____

_____

_____

_____

Case Study #12

Marion Beck is a frail elderly woman, 87 years of age with moderate dementia.

She has a history of osteoarthritis, back pain and knee pains.

Currently she takes MEslon, 15 mg po q12h for past four months.

In the last several days, she had become very agitated, refusing food and resisting care. Marion no longer recognizes RCAs who she normally knows. She is paranoid that someone is coming to get her and starting to refuse medications, saying they are poison.

10. Explain the potential implications of these changes in her behavior. _____

_____

_____

_____

11. Give details of what you report to the physician. _____

_____

_____

_____

12. Describe supportive comfort measures you could implement immediately. _____

_____

_____

_____

_____

12. What do you believe might be of concern to the family?

_____

_____

13. If you identify delirium, would it be appropriate to investigate the cause? Why or why not? _____

_____

14. If it is not appropriate to investigate the causes, what medications might be useful for palliation? See the Fraser Health website for suggestions. _____

_____

_____

_____

Small and Large Group Discussions (Time permitting)

15. Discuss the Case #11 and #12 in light of the importance of involving patients as much as possible in deciding treatment plan._____

_____

_____

_____

16. Identify the challenges of delirium for family members._____

_____

_____

_____

_____

17. If either person were in the home, what do you need to provide for the family in order for them to respond to the changing needs? e.g. contact information for 24/7. ____

_____

_____

_____

_____

Last Days and Hours

Beliefs and Baggage

1. Describe your experience with caring for someone through to death. _____

_____

_____

_____

2. Describe your beliefs about dying. _____

_____

_____

_____

3. Describe your beliefs about death. _____

_____

_____

_____

4. We sometimes hear people say that it is a privilege to be with a person when they die. Reflect on this and write your thoughts about why this might be? _____

_____

_____

_____

5. We sometimes hear people say that they do not want to be on shift when their patients die. Reflect on this and write your thoughts about why this might be? _____

_____

_____

_____

6. Explain your feelings about family involvement and visiting near time of death. _____

_____

_____

_____

_____

7. We sometimes hear people say, "No one should die alone" or more recently we are starting to hear "People like to die alone." What are your thoughts about these different opinions? _____

_____

_____

_____

8. What are your beliefs about "religion" and "spirituality"? How might this influence the care you provide? _____

_____

_____

_____

_____

Concepts and Content

Short Answer Questions

9. Planning for care through to death involves access to resources and support. What could this look like in the community where you live or work? _____

_____

_____

_____

_____

10. Families may ask "When will death occur?" or "How long does s/he have?" – Explain some of the reasons for this question. _____

_____

_____

_____

_____

_____

_____

11. Describe 3 strategies and include examples of questions that you would ask, to assist family to understand that death is nearing. _____

_____

_____

_____

_____

_____

_____

_____

_____

_____

_____

Dying with Chronic Illness

12. Why is it challenging to prognosticate for people dying with chronic illness? _____

_____

_____

_____

_____

13. What might a person miss if they do not realize they are dying? What might family miss if they do not realize the patient is dying?_____

_____

_____

_____

_____

_____

_____

_____

14. List five sentinel events that may indicate that death is imminent for persons dying with late stage dementia. _____

_____

_____

_____

Psychosocial Implications of Physical Changes

15. For each of the physical changes that may occur in the last days and hours, identify i) one psychosocial implication for the family, and ii) one comfort measure for the patient.

a. Increased drowsiness - i)_____

_____

ii) _____

_____

b. Reduced intake - i) _____

_____

ii) _____

_____

c. Confusion and restlessness - i) _____

_____

ii) _____

_____

d. Difficulty swallowing - i) _____

_____

ii) _____

_____

e. Unresponsiveness - i) _____

_____

ii) _____

_____

f. Changes in breathing sounds - i) _____

_____

ii) _____

_____

g. Changes in skin colour and temperature - i)_____

_____

ii) _____

_____

h. Twitching - i) _____

_____

ii) _____

_____

i. Eyes, open or closed - i) _____

_____

ii) _____

_____

j. Bowel and bladder - i) _____

_____

ii) _____

_____

k. Breathing and expression at time of death - i) _____

_____

ii) _____

_____

Integration and Application

16. Discuss and debrief the Content and Concepts questions.

17. You are assigned to pronounce death. What physical assessment needs to be completed? _____

_____

18. Who needs to be notified? _____

_____

19. What needs to be documented after death? _____

_____

_____

_____

20. What other policies may be present in a facility regarding care of the body following death? _____

_____

_____

21. Following death in a facility it is necessary to clean the room and prepare for the next admission. This can be uncomfortable for both the nurse and the family/loved ones. How would you identify needs of the family before starting to clear/clean the room? ____

_____

_____

_____

_____

22. If you are involved in collecting and storing personal effects and valuables, there will be a policy to follow. What might this policy include? _____

_____

_____

_____

_____

_____

23. Describe current health authority policy on LPN/RN pronouncement of death. _____

_____

_____

_____

24. Provide key details about local or provincial policies on *Expected Death* (e.g. BC's/ Ontario's recent document "Expected Death Form")._____

_____

_____

_____

_____

_____

Large Group Discussions

Refer to nursing texts for procedures on caring for the body following death (postmortem care).

25. Are these procedures current practices in the settings in your local facilities or community?_____

_____

_____

_____

26. What is expected following death in your local facilities? _____

_____

_____

_____

_____

_____

_____

Case Study #13

Susan Linton is 46 years old with end stage cardiac disease, has shown a slow and steady decline over past few weeks. She appears to be in her last days. PPS 20%, unable to swallow, no longer taking foods. Family are concerned about the decreased intake, and worried about dehydration.

27. What signs would you assess if Susan is uncomfortable without fluid intake? _____

_____

_____

_____

28. What are comfort measures that may help Susan be more comfortable without providing artificial hydration? _____

_____

_____

_____

Susan is no longer able to take her oral medications. She currently takes:

MEslon 30mg *po q12* hours

Ativan 1 mg *sl q8h* prn for restlessness

Haldol 1 mg *po* at *hs* for nausea

Cardiac medications

29. Which medications could be discontinued? _____

_____

_____

30. Which medication(s) could be offered by another route and continued through to
death? _____

_____

_____

Role Play

31. Susan's family is concerned about what they might expect in the coming days.
Describe your role in this discussion with Susan's family. _____

_____

_____

_____

_____

32. Describe strategies that you might suggest to the family to help them provide
comfort, and to feel comfort themselves. _____

_____

_____

_____

_____

_____

Supporting Children Living with Dying
Beliefs and Baggage

1. Describe your most significant (or "first") experience with death as a child, including thoughts and feelings that you might recall. _____

_____

_____

_____

2. What do you recall were the beliefs that your parents/caregivers held about children and death?_____

_____

_____

_____

3. Describe your current beliefs about children being told about a loved one's impending death. _____

_____

_____

_____

4. Describe your current beliefs about a child's involvement in funerals and burials._____

_____

_____

_____

_____

Concepts and Content

5. List and explain the rationale behind ten guidelines for talking to a child about the death of a parent/loved one. _____

_____

_____

_____

_____

_____

_____

_____

_____

_____

6. Describe three concerns children are likely to have when a parent is dying. _____

_____

_____

_____

_____

_____

Integration and Application

Case Study #14

You are working with an eight year old whose mother is dying of breast cancer. The child knows that her mother has cancer, but has not been told that she will die from it.

7. The child's parents have asked the nursing team to provide them with information on how to talk to their child. What are some principles that you might offer the team? _____

_____

_____

_____

_____

_____

_____

_____

_____

_____

_____

_____

_____

Rituals
Beliefs and Baggage

1. Explain your beliefs about the role of rituals in your life and describe any rituals surrounding death that are comforting to you._____

_____

_____

_____

_____

_____

2. Are there any rituals that you might feel uncomfortable with as death nears? _____

_____

_____

_____

_____

_____

3. Reflect on how to integrate and honour the rituals of patients/families if they differ from your own. _____

_____

_____

_____

_____

Concepts and Content

Short Answer Questions

4. Define the term "ritual." _____

_____

_____

5. Whose goals do death rituals meet? _____

_____

_____

6. List 5 rituals associated with death and explain their meaning. _____

_____

_____

_____

_____

7. Describe the strategies and practices you use to demonstrate respect for the body following death. _____

_____

_____

_____

_____

Integration and Application

8. As you welcome Irene to the unit describe the information you could offer, and what you could include in a tour of the unit to increase her comfort? _____

_____

_____

9. Interdisciplinary, inter-professional care is one of the "essentials" in HPC. What contacts in the care team might be helpful for this family?_____

_____

_____

_____

_____

10. What resources in your local community might be helpful for Irene? e.g. local hospice? bereavement support groups? chaplain? _____

_____

_____

_____

9. Describe 3 resources available through Canadian Virtual Hospice that you feel would be useful to someone who is dying or caregiving._____

_____

_____

_____

_____

10. Describe resources this site might offer you._____

_____

_____

_____

_____

On Being Up Close
and Personal with the Dying

The Psychosocial Perspective
Beliefs and Baggage

1. Think back to a time when you felt "seen, heard and validated." Describe the feelings you experienced at that time. What was this impact of this experience?

Alternatively, if you cannot remember a specific positive experience, think of a time when you felt that your ideas and feelings or input were discredited or ignored. Describe the feelings you experienced at that time. _____

_____

_____

_____

_____

_____

2. Explain the risks as you perceive them, when you go beyond "just focusing on the task at hand" and instead you "see and respond" to the whole person before you. _____

_____

_____

_____

_____

_____

Concepts and Content

Short Answer Questions

3. Give 2 examples that demonstrate your understanding of how the psychosocial perspective might affect how you provide physical care. _____

_____

_____

_____

_____

_____

4. Explain your understanding of why healing is different from curing._____

_____

_____

_____

Integration and Application

Small and Large Group Discussions

5. Discuss answers to the questions in Concepts and Content.

6. Why is it important to learn the art of "being with" people? Give an example from your caregiving that illustrates "doing" and "being" at the same time. _____

_____

_____

_____

_____

_____

_____

_____

_____

_____

7. If you were ill and dying, what would be the 5 most important things that you would want caregivers to do, know, or remember?

Share your list with a colleague and compare lists. Reflect on the lists and write about what you learned.

_____

_____

_____

_____

_____

_____

_____

_____

_____

_____

_____

The Dance
Beliefs and Baggage

1. Describe the words and images that come to mind when you think of your own "family dance." _____

_____

_____

_____

_____

2. Compare your family dance to any others you may know about and describe differences that are visible. _____

_____

_____

_____

_____

_____

3. What do you value in your own "dance"? What, if anything, is missing? _____

_____

_____

_____

_____

_____

Concepts and Contents

4. Summarize "The Dance" and its relationship to the concept of boundaries._____

_____

_____

_____

_____

_____

5. List 3 things that you can do when you stay on the *edge* of someone else's dance floor.

_____

_____

_____

_____

_____

6. What is lost when you don't stay on the edge of the patient's/family's dance floor?

_____

_____

_____

_____

7. Explain what "therapeutic distance" means._____

_____

_____

_____

_____

8. Why are personal awareness and clarity important to maintaining a therapeutic distance? _____

_____

_____

_____

_____

9. What are the 3 cues that let us know that we have "crossed the line" onto another person's dance floor? _____

_____

_____

_____

_____

10. What is a "hook" in the context of the image of the dance? _____

_____

_____

_____

11) What are three things you can do to remain clear about boundaries in your work?

_____

_____

_____

_____

Integration and Application

12. Discuss your answers to Concepts and Contents questions with the larger group.

13. Describe any "hooks" that might take you onto someone else's dance floor. _____

_____

_____

_____

_____

_____

_____

14. Describe a time when you crossed a boundary onto someone else's dance floor. Why did you do it? What was lost or gained?_____

_____

_____

_____

15. What supports and nourishes you in your own dance that helps you maintain boundaries in your work? _____

_____

_____

_____

_____

Case Study #16

An older man is dying in hospital. The daughter (who lives in the same town and has always been there to help her parents) and the man's wife are in his room. Another daughter (who moved back east to raise her family) has just arrived, wants to know what's happening and appears to be trying to take charge. The two daughters are arguing over their father's bed while their mother sits quietly in the corner.

Small and Large Group Discussions

16. Describe how you might you intervene while still respecting their family dance. _____

_____

_____

_____

_____

_____

_____

_____

Principles in Building Therapeutic Relationships
Beliefs and Baggage

1. Describe distractions that would be most likely to interfere with your ability to be fully present with patients and families._____

_____

_____

_____

_____

2. Write about personal challenges that you would face in an encounter with a patient or family member who had different values, beliefs or coping styles than yours. Give 2 examples. _____

_____

_____

_____

_____

_____

_____

_____

_____

Concepts and Content

3. List 5 principles in building a therapeutic (healthy) relationships (Essentials, pg 140). ___

_____

_____

_____

_____

Integration and Application

4. How can you demonstrate "respect and a willingness to learn" to a patient and/or family that you had just met? Share your ideas with a colleague and discuss the similarities and differences in your choices.

_____

_____

_____

_____

_____

_____

_____

_____

Communication Skills
Beliefs and Baggage

1. Describe the way that you normally communicate stress, anger, frustration, joy, and/or sadness? Include verbal and nonverbal methods. _____

_____

_____

_____

_____

2. Explain how you usually respond when other people express these emotions. _____

_____

_____

3. Think of a time when someone you know was struggling with a problem or was sad. Describe how you felt. _____

_____

_____

4. How important was it to you to find a solution or "make it all OK?" What happened?_

_____

_____

_____

5. Describe your comfort level with the concept of "creating a safe and sacred place for grief to be expressed." _____

_____

_____

_____

_____

_____

6. What would need to change to increase your comfort level? _____

_____

_____

_____

_____

_____

Concepts and Content

Short Answer Questions

7. List 5 reasons that explain why open-ended questions facilitate good communication.

_____

_____

_____

_____

8. List 4 open-ended questions. _____

_____

_____

_____

_____

9. Explain how you know when someone is really listening to you. _____

_____

_____

_____

_____

10. Define in your own words the "Fix-it trap." _____

_____

_____

_____

_____

11. How would you know if you were in the "Fix-it trap." _____

_____

_____

_____

_____

12. Explain why the "Fix-it trap" contributes to the tendency to label patients and families.

_____

_____

_____

13. What are three roadblocks to good communication and what question(s) do you need to ask for each one? _____

_____

_____

_____

_____

_____

_____

_____

_____

_____

Integration and Application

Pairs Exercise and Group Discussion

14. For this exercise work in groups of two. If there is an extra individual, work in a group of three. Prepare to discuss experience with the large group.

- Partner #1 - Share a problem (real or imagined) with Partner #2.

- Partner #2 - Listen and respond with open-ended questions and phrases such as "Tell me more about that."

- At the same time however, listen to you own inner "talk" about wanting to "fix the problem" by suggesting solutions, minimizing the discomfort or reassuring your partner that "everything will work out."

15. Debrief by writing about your experience in the exercise. _____

_____

_____

_____

_____

_____

_____

_____

_____

16. Switch roles and repeat the entire exercise. Debrief by writing about your experience in the exercise. _____

_____

_____

_____

_____

_____

17. Share your results with the large group in the form of an answer to the following two questions:

- What did it feel like to be listened to without being 'fixed'?
- What did it feel like to just listen and not try to solve the problem?

18. After the large group discussion, write about your feelings during the experience and the knowledge you gained with this experience. Specifically, are there any changes that you will make when listening to patients and family? _____

_____

_____

_____

_____

_____

_____

_____

_____

_____

_____

_____

_____

_____

The Nature of Grief
Beliefs and Baggage

1. Think of a time when your family or friends shared an experience of loss. Describe how individuals experienced and expressed their grief differently. _____

_____

_____

_____

_____

2. Think about your comfort level with people who grieve differently than you. What do you believe would increase your comfort level? _____

_____

_____

_____

Concepts and Content

3. Define "loss." _____

_____

4. Define "grief." _____

_____

5. Define "transitions." _____

_____

_____

4. Using the body map indicate with arrows and labels, **8** ways that a person might be affected by grief (e.g. you might indicate 'forgetfulness' by drawing an arrow to the head and labeling it).

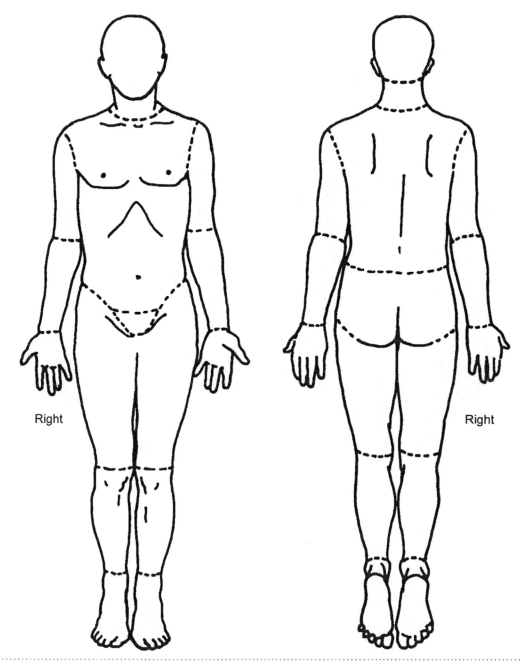

Right

Right

5. Draw on the body map where grief touches you.

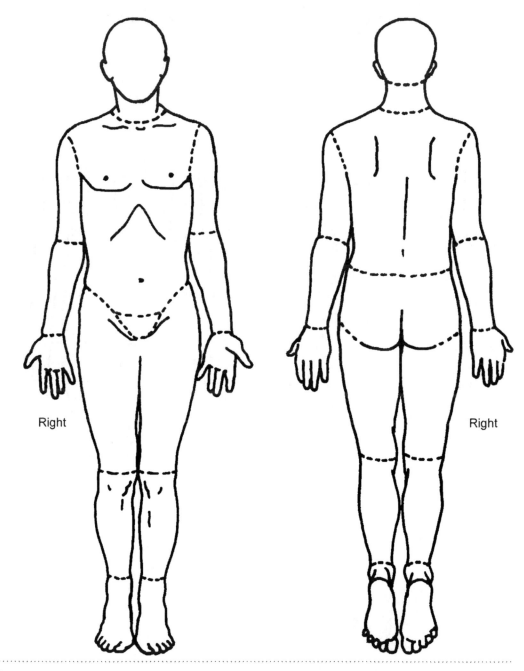

Right

Right

6. Explain the statement "dying often involves a series of losses." Give 3 examples of possible losses. _____

_____

_____

_____

_____

_____

7. Describe the potential effects of grief on a patient's or family member's ability to receive information or make decisions. _____

_____

_____

_____

_____

_____

_____

_____

_____

_____

_____

_____

Integration and Application

8. Five things I would want caregivers to do or know when I am dying.

1. _____

   _____

2. _____

   _____

3. _____

   _____

4. _____

   _____

5. _____

   _____

Pairs Exercise

9. Materials: 4 small pieces of paper for each participant, pen or pencil.

Part A

   1. Write one activity you enjoy doing on each piece of paper. (4 pieces of paper/ 4 activities).
   2. Turn the pieces of paper upside down with the writing facing the floor.
   3. Fan the pieces of paper out and let your partner choose two to take from you.
   4. Notice what you have lost (i.e. bowling and swimming).

Part B

   1. Now imagine that your physician has just told you that because of the progression of your 'disease', you can no longer do the two things that were just taken away from you by your partner.
   2. Share with your partner your feelings about the following two questions:

- The **series of losses** that are involved with the loss of each activity (e.g. bowling, exercise, social interaction, identity as a quilter, baker etc).
- Your **first reaction** to being told that you can no longer do the two activities that were taken away.

3. Have the facilitator write down the participants' first reactions to this loss as they call them out.

4. Review the list from the perspective that while all the responses are "normal" reactions to loss, how often do we label patient and family responses as:
   - "….the patient/family member who is angry about their ongoing losses as the difficult patient/family member"
   - "….the patient who is terrified of what lies ahead as someone who doesn't cope well" or
   - "….the person who is in 'denial', who won't 'face the facts' like they 'should,' as someone who is weak".

5. Discuss these ideas in the large group:
   - How does making judgments about how other people react to loss, get in the way of compassionate care?
   - How would you want to be treated if you were experiencing the loss of a loved one or of your own health?
   - Why is it important to be aware of our own grieving style(s), (what is normal for us) in order to maintain a therapeutic distance in our relationship with patients and families?

_____

_____

_____

_____

_____

_____

_____

_____

10. Describe what might account for the difference in Abigail's behaviour between the night shift and the day shift._____

_____

_____

_____

11. What questions do you need to ask the PATIENT, your teammates and the family? ___

_____

_____

_____

12. Is this a pattern, or is this unusual? Explain.

_____

_____

_____

_____

_____

Self Care and the Recovery Cycle

Beliefs and Baggage

1. Think about how you care for yourself. Do you care for yourself as well as you care for others? Why or why not? _____

_____

_____

_____

_____

_____

_____

2. What personal beliefs, attitudes or opinions interfere with your ability to commit to regular self care? _____

_____

_____

_____

_____

_____

3. What are the signs that let you know you're "running on fumes", such as when you feel tired, stressed, overworked or unappreciated? _____

_____

_____

_____

_____

4. What do you do when you feel like this? How does it affect your work? How does it affect your relationships? _____

_____

_____

_____

_____

_____

5. When was the last time that you deliberately engaged in self care. Why? What did you do? How did it make you feel? _____

_____

_____

_____

_____

Concepts and Content

6. The Recovery Cycle is a model for strength training and injury prevention for athletes. What are your thoughts in applying this model to caregivers? _____

_____

_____

_____

_____

7. Essentials refers to "Relaxation, Meditation, and Revelation" as the steps in Recovery. Explain how these concepts fit within your own philosophy of self care. _____

_____

_____

_____

_____

_____

_____

8. Describe alternative strategies that you would implement in the recovery cycle instead.

_____

_____

_____

_____

9. What does "overcompensation" or "full recovery" feel like for you? _____

_____

_____

_____

10. What gets in the way of you doing "self care" and rebuilding in time for recovery?

_____

_____

_____

11. Describe the relationship between our ability to care for ourselves and our ability to care for others. _____

_____

_____

_____

12. List 3 common obstacles to self care. _____

_____

_____

_____

13. Describe 3 self care ideas from the manual and then add 3 ideas of your own._____

_____

_____

_____

_____

_____

_____

_____

_____

Integration and Application

Group Activity

14. Materials: magazines, scissors, glue, marking pens and 11"x14" construction paper, preferably in a variety of colours.

Directions: In small groups cut out pictures, words, slogans etc from the magazines and spread them out on a large surface.

Address the following questions in the collage:

1.   Who am I ?
2.   What do I long for? and
3.   What do I love? (What nourishes me and sustains me)

You can create three collages or combine all questions on one collage.

Allow time for participants to go the pictures/words etc and choose as many as they want. They can combine all three questions on one collage or do a separate collage for each question.

Large Group Discussion

Each person who wants to can take 4-5 minutes to talk about their collage and their process of making it.

For example, you might share:

*   What was easy/difficult or fun/challenging about this exercise?

*   What surprised you about what your answers?

*   Do you spend as much time as you want with the people/things you cherish? Why/ why not?

- Who is responsible for seeing that you get more of what you need in your life?

- What if anything is preventing you from doing something you want to do before you die?

- What is one thing you could do right now to nurture that dream and bring it to fruition?

Resources from Life and Death Matters

Visit the store at www.lifeanddeathmatters.ca to purchase resources

Essentials in Hospice Palliative Care - 2nd Edition

Written by Katherine Murray

This manual is an excellent resource for palliative caregivers - including family, community health workers, resident care assistants, nurses and anyone wanting a solid easy to read foundation in caring for people who are dying.
ISBN 978-0-9739828-1-7

Essentials in Hospice Palliative Care Workbook
Study Guide for Nurses

Written by Katherine Murray

A study guide to accompany the Essentials in Hospice Palliative Care text, written specifically for nurses. Engaging, practical and reflective activities based on the Essentials in Hospice Palliative Care manual. Designed to reinforce learning and integration of new concepts.
ISBN 978-0-9739828-2-4

Essentials in Hospice Palliative Care Workbook
Study Guide for Health Care Workers

Written by Katherine Murray

A study guide to accompany the Essentials in Hospice Palliative Care text, written specifically for health care workers. Designed to reinforce learning and integration of new concepts.
ISBN 978-0-9739828-2-8

Reflections in Hospice Palliative Care - A Personal Writing Journal

This reflective writing journal contains thought-provoking writing stems designed to assist individuals to integrate theory with practice.
ISBN 978-0-9739828-3-1

Essentials in Hospice Palliative Care Videos

Introduction to Managing Pain

In a role play with a "family member" Kath Murray shares principles of pain management, explaining palliative strategies, dispelling myths about opioids and encouraging the development of comfort measures that are tailor-made to the patient.
ISBN 978-0-9739828-6-2

Managing Dyspnea

Kath Murray presents an overview of dyspnea, that includes how to recognize, assess and manage dyspnea, as well as comfort measures to support individuals experiencing dyspnea. ISBN 978-0-9739828-7-9

Boundaries and Self Care
Elizabeth Causton addresses the risks of becoming "like family" and the benefits of maintaining therapeutic boundaries with clients as a form of self care. ISBN 978-0-9739828-8-6

Essentials in Hospice Palliative Care Teaching Series
This PowerPoint© series was developed by Kath to support educators in teaching "essentials in hospice palliative care". Designed in conjunction with the manual and workbook, these visual presentations are ready-to-use and can also be adapted to local needs. ISBN 978-0-9739828-5-5

Visit the store at www.lifeanddeathmatters.ca to purchase resources

Join us for online education at www.LDMonline.ca
Enhance your capacity to provide care for the dying and bereaved while exploring current issues and hot topics in death and dying in this comprehensive online hospice palliative care program. Courses are completed in approximately 10 hours over a 3 week period. Open ended registration allows participants to begin any month! Take one course or take them all and complete your certificate.

Each course features a captivating mix of readings, assignments and/or field trips, and fosters the development of a dynamic online learning community with discussion forums, teleconferences, guest speakers and chats. Work online with facilitators and participants around the globe in a creative fun environment, integrating theory and knowledge into practice in your personal and professional life.

LaVergne, TN USA
14 February 2010
172975LV00003B/3/P